LORD, THE TIGER IN MY TANK IS CANCER

How I Survived the Surprise Birthday Gift

Marlene Marshall

Copyright © 2021 by Marlene Marshall

All rights reserved. This book or any portion thereof may not be reproduced or used in any manner whatsoever without the express written permission of the publisher except for the use of brief quotations in a book review.

Printed in the United States of America

ISBN: 9798521987566

Cover Design: Shakira (Kira) Marshall
kiradivine@gmail.com

Contact Information
Marlene Marshall
msquared7@aol.com

In Loving Memory of My Parents:
Emil And Idaliah Monsanto
and a Dear Friend:
Marguerite D Nonni

Dedication

To my husband, the love of my life, my greatest supporter and my rock. He has encouraged me through this journey to share my testimony. Thank you from the bottom of my heart.

To my daughter, Shakira (Kira) who has been pushing me to write as she believes that I have a lot to share. I hope that you learn that depending on God and constantly praying he will always light your path as you build your future. Use the gifts that he bestowed on you, share with others and remember that it was my faith that brought me thus far and it is faith in the Almighty that will raise you above every storm you encounter.

To my cousin Ingrid Bryan who is currently starting on the journey I just completed. Know that it was Faith that brought me through. Place your faith in the God of Love and Mercy, believe and all will be well.

And last but not least to my friends Dianne, Kamala and Marlyn my circle of strong women, thank you for your love, support, wisdom and encouragement. You were there through the whole process I pray that God will continue to richly bless you and your family.

Table of Contents

Acknowledgments ix

Foreword xi

Introduction 1

Chapter 1 - What is Endometrial Cancer (Uterine Cancer) 3

Chapter 2 - The Diagnosis 7

Chapter 3 - Reaction After Consultation 13

Chapter 4 - The Surprise 17

Chapter 5: The Surprise Party 21

Chapter 6: Phase 1 and 2 Action Plans 25

Chapter 7: Obtaining a Support System and Seeking Spiritual Counsel 31

Chapter 8 - The First Visit To The Infusion Center 35

Chapter 9 - Phase 3 and Final Stage of Treatment 41

Chapter 10 - Medications and Other Aids 47

Ways To Learn More 51

Food Suggestions 52

References That Helped Me on This Journey 56

Acknowledgments

Thank you, Vanessa Collins, my writing coach. You believed in me, you encouraged me in your gentle but firm way because you knew that there was someone out there waiting for this information and the mission of my message. I really needed that push.

To my daughter, Shakira (Kira) Marshall, I told you what my vision was for the cover of my book and you created and tweaked it until we came up with the final product. Thank you for your creativity.

Foreword

As we journey through life traversing the unknown in search of our destiny, we know not the moment nor the hour when the speed bumps of life will hit or the random attacks of nature's wild algorithm will happen, regardless we carry faith, hope and courage in our stash. By design we carry the audacity of hope with us for we thrive and survive with these driving factors, pushing us to our highest potential and sometimes beyond our breaking point. It is in these moments of crisis when our faith and strength are put to the ultimate test, a life exam of sorts that one can only prepare for unknowingly through the trials and struggles of life. Like iron forged through the fires of strife and sadness, we continue to press forward knowing that God promised us that troubles last not always. "Weeping may endure for a night, but joy cometh in the morning" Psalm 30:5.

Unwavering Faith

Like the popular George Michael song entitled "Faith", author Marlene Marshall artfully exhibits its undeniable presence through her journey. In the song there is a repetitive emphasis on the word faith and just how much of it "I gotta have faith f-faith f-faith f-faith". Unwavering faith is a tool most people utilize in every phase of their life's journey. We all utilize elements of faith to navigate our daily lives as human beings. When you plant a seed, it is with hope and faith that you watch it grow (along with water, sun and lots of TLC*). There are many examples of moments in life where hope and faith are hand in hand working together to create and manifest one's desired outcome. Marlene Marshall's unwavering faith is quite evident as she takes us through battling Endometrial cancer. What the Tiger may not have known is that her tank is filled with unwavering faith.

Support Systems

We've all heard the sayings: "It takes a village to raise a child" an African proverb that points to the significance of community in one's development. Or "Your network is your net worth" which is a phrase that reflects the power and value of relationships. One of my favorite Guyanese creolize patois idioms "One, one dutty build dam" which translates to little by little we can build something large by working together. All of these sayings in one way or another point to the value of community and the importance of having a strong support system often referred to as our "inner-circle". Who's in your circle? Have you taken the time to re-evaluate your circle recently? Friends are people we choose to associate with and are therefore chosen family and let's be honest, not all of our family members make the cut for access to our inner circle. We choose our circle and surround ourselves with like-minded individuals who reflect common values, lifestyles, sense of humor, religious beliefs, personality traits, etc. Sometimes we don't choose our circle as God places people in our lives for a reason and/or a season that we may not have chosen otherwise.

In times of crises, we undoubtedly turn to those closest to us in hopes of receiving unconditional love and support. Friends and family create the safety net we all require from time to time, holding us up in our times of need. These moments we all face in life, force us to lean on our loved ones and exemplifies just how important it is to have a network of supporters. We also lean on the expertise, guidance and knowledge of the healthcare professionals and traditional cultural home remedies alike. Marshall paints a narrative showing how she used these tools of unwavering faith and an unbreakable support system to guide and protect her through this journey into the unknown. Of course, no journey could be complete without the sole and utter guidance of the Almighty.

Kira Divine

Introduction

I grew up in a British Colony and church was an integral part of my life. I remember thinking that one day I could be a Nun. I think that was because the nuns at Church of the Holy Rosary took great care of the children in the parish and community. Years later I ended up working in Social Services and used my educational background to nurture and counsel youths.

Have you ever been faced with a situation that you thought would never come your way? Over the years I heard of many friends, acquaintances, neighbors, family and friends who went through fighting cancer. Some of them never recovered. To me it was the dreaded illness, one that I would not wish on anyone. It is under these circumstances that you fight with your faith and sometimes lose hope, but it is also a time to find your inner strength, faith, courage, humility and you fight back with all the might and strength trusting in the Almighty to allow you to be a miracle. It is because of my having to walk through the fire that I decided to share my story.

It is my hope that whoever reads my story will find the faith and strength, if faced with the same journey that they place all in the hands of the Almighty to overcome the obstacles that will be thrown their way.

It is also my hope that you receive the best medical care so that your chances of survival would be a successful one. Early detection is key.

Chapter 1 - What is Endometrial Cancer (Uterine Cancer)

There are five known gynecologic cancers: Cervical, Ovarian, Uterine, Vaginal, and Vulva. My book will concentrate on Endometrial Cancer also known as Uterine cancer. Endometrial cancer is the most common gynecological Cancer in the United States.

As per the American Cancer Society they do not exactly know what causes most cases of Endometrial cancer but there are risk factors strongly linked to this type of cancer like obesity, hormone imbalance, bleeding during menopause and after menopause.

Having knowledge of this can definitely make a difference in your survival rate. One of the most dominant warnings is bleeding during and after menopause. You should get checked out by your gynecologist as soon as you see these signs.

It is often best to not dismiss this sign but question what is wrong with your body before it develops into something more serious.

The cancer cells developed has estrogen and or progesterone receptors on their surfaces. The receptors and hormones interact and cause increase growth of the Endometrium.

As the growth increases it becomes more and more abnormal until it develops into cancer. It appears that not only does this cancer affect the balance between our estrogen and progesterone, but our DNA of certain genes cause some of the changes.

Research on Endometrial cancer is being done in medical centers around the world to help in early detection and treatment. Of course, like any other illness early detection is imperative and key to a favorable outcome. Treatment for this kind of cancer is as per scientist in a clinical trial and should be considered for anyone diagnosed and in any stage of Endometrial cancer.

I am not a scientist, but I had no idea that such a cancer existed until I was diagnosed then I was forced to read the literature given me by my doctor, along with researching the internet and Google to get a better understanding of what was happening to my body.

Our bodies undergo not only hormonal changes, but gene changes and these changes contribute to the medical crises we face in our lives. If the scientist can find a way to detect endometrial cancer early or before it develops perhaps it can be stopped before it becomes cancer.

We have to pay attention to the changes in our bodies and talk to our doctors. If you are not comfortable with the doctor's advice you can always seek a second opinion, after all your health is important.

Reflections

Chapter 2 - The Diagnosis

It was a beautiful evening in December of 2017, and I was looking forward to attend my friends annual New Year's Eve celebration. This was a fun party with mature guests who had been friends over the years. The company was good, and the food was even better.

My husband and I knew the family for about 42 years. We shared in many challenges with our children, our jobs, church, illness and involvement in the different group activities in the church and the community, anyhow at this joyful gathering I observed something strange in my body functioning when I used the bathroom and it alarmed me. I took care of myself and proceeded to enjoy the party keeping in mind to contact my doctor as soon as the holidays were over.

The next available business day I called my doctor and she advised me as I was out of town that I should go to the nearest walk-in clinic and ask them to examine me and to forward the results of any tests that they run on me to her office. I followed my doctor's instructions.

I went to the local pharmacy and logged into their intake computer listing my complaints and symptoms and I had to list my insurance coverage in order to be seen. I had to now sit and wait for a nurse or NP to call me.

In about twenty minutes I was called by the nurse who went over my information. She took my pressure, temperature, pulse and asked me to give her a urine specimen. The nurse then gave me a prescription for some pills, and she advised me to follow up with my doctor. I requested that she send the report of the tests to my doctor in my hometown. She never addressed the health crisis that I was facing at that moment.

I waited three days and then I called my doctor's office to see whether she had received the results and to schedule an appointment with her but to my surprise I was told that she was out of the office sick and that I would have to call her office in three weeks. I called again and the receptionist informed me that the doctor was still out ill, and they did not know when she would return. I was concerned since not only did the pharmacy clinic not call me but now I could not see my primary care physician.

I felt that there was some urgency for me to see a doctor as my body was not functioning the way it should, so I called the gynecologist. Hallelujah!! he listened to my symptoms, and he immediately scheduled me to see him on January 25, 2018. I was relieved. I could now get to the bottom of what was causing all this trouble in my tank.

I kept my appointment, and he quickly took some blood, urine, pap smear and a complete vaginal examination. He explained to me that my symptoms could mean nothing or something, but he was happy that I was paying attention to my body as that would prove to be a plus in the early detection of what was wrong.

The next day I received a call from the Doctor's office. He informed me that my pap test was good, but the blood and urine work up was in question and he wanted me to see a specialist so that he could go over the findings and have a consultation with me.

He gave me a list of three top Gynecological Oncologist, and I immediately called and scheduled the appointment.

On February 6th I consulted with the specialist and on February 7, 2018, I was diagnosed with Endometrial Cancer (Uterine).

In consultation the doctor said to me, "We cannot sit on this, it is crucial that I immediately schedule you for a hysterectomy, after that a battery of chemotherapy followed by radiation. Today we will go ahead and schedule the hysterectomy and get you prepared for this first phase of treatment as soon as possible.

Could you imagine what a punch that was to my stomach. This was devastatingly sad news. There was no time to digest my situation. I said a few silent prayers and let the doctor go ahead and schedule me for emergency major surgery.

Reflections

Cancer attacks when least expected so are you paying attention to your body?

_____

_____

How are you listening to your body?

_____

_____

_____

Do you believe that God warns you of impending danger? How should you respond?

_____

_____

_____

How would you have reacted had you experienced the same warning signs?

_____

_____

_____

_____

_____

_____

_____

Do you ever take time out to listen to that still small voice each day of your life?

_____

_____

_____

_____

Chapter 3 - Reaction After Consultation

Unknown to me my family was planning some kind of celebration for my birthday. Little did they know that my birthday gift was the diagnosis of Endometrial Cancer.

How was I to be happy and celebrate with family on this milestone of my life? God in his promise was blessing me with three score and ten years. He would not bring me to this point of his promise having every hope of enjoying additional blessings going forward only to be diagnosed with something that could take me out. It was like being at the cusp of the tree of life in full bloom then only to fizzle out. What a Birthday gift?

So, this is the tiger in my tank.

It was as if everything was coming at me. How was I going to share this serious problem that I was facing with my immediate family? I immediately fell on my knees and prayed and prayed and yes, I questioned God and of course asked him why.

Why me? Did I not try hard enough to live up to your expectations? How did I fail you Lord? Will you walk with me through the fire and save me like you saved "Shadrach, Meshach and Abednego," or Jonah and all the others you saved.? Who do I let know what I was about to face? and how would I be able to balance it all? And what about my future? I knew that I had not completed my purpose/mission here on earth.

There is so much more to do with very little time to do it all and so I began to torture myself; with my mind racing and I felt caught in a sandstorm and there was no way to hide or find shelter until the storm blew over. Who would extend their hands and pull me back to reality? After a few moments of quite I realized that God had given me all the tools to work through this test. Wow! This was just a test and at that moment I recalled what Jesus said to the woman with the issue of blood "Thy faith had made thee whole," (Matthew 9:22) and he said this again and again in Luke (17:19), Luke 18:42, Matthew 8:13 and Matthew 15:28.

Faith is linked to healing then I must have faith to overcome what was ahead of me.

Reflections

What do you think "The Tiger In My Tank" refers to in this narrative?

_____

_____

_____

_____

_____

How else would you describe it? Give examples below.

_____

_____

_____

_____

_____

Have you ever encountered inner conflict and fear? If yes, where and who did you turn to for support?

_____

_____

_____

_____

_____

_____

_____

_____

_____

_____

_____

_____

Chapter 4 - The Surprise

I had been so busy running around setting up doctor's appointments that several family members had arrived in town. I had been looking to a February 14th outing with my daughter. As a birthday gift she had secured tickets to Carnegie Hall to a concert with one of her favorite stage performers, jazz musician Gregory Porter and that was also on my mind.

I wondered whether I would start to feel any different even though my surgery date was not set up yet. So many clues that should have alerted me that something special was afoot, and I did not detect anything.

So, my daughter calls me from a dress boutique and she says, "Mom which of these dresses do you like?" I gave her my choice and she said, "I like that one too, I will see you later." and she hung up. I quickly forgot the incident since the doctor had given me a lot of literature to read which I did read as I prepared dinner. I was feeling good so far just annoyed that I had to be wearing a protective pad which made me feel that my teenage years had started over again only this time there seemed to be no break in the discomfort.

A few days later my daughter tells me that the family will be taking me out Saturday for my birthday. They will be taking me to a new exclusive restaurant and since it was my special day, I had to dress elegantly then she pulls out a gorgeous dark gray shimmering cocktail gown and she said, "Mom try this on." It was the same dress she had asked me about a week earlier when she called me from the Dress Boutique. "This is the dress you are wearing on Saturday mom. Oh! By the way, you must be ready by 3:00 pm."

I was in no mood for fussing, so I tried on the dress, and it was a perfect fit except for the length and being a little loose. Then she says, "Mom it will work. It is one-of-a-kind dress, and this is the only one in stock. It is beautiful I will take it to the cleaners and have them alter the hem they only have to cut about three inches and you will not know the difference."

I left her up to her ploys since all this could have been avoided if she had invited me shopping and I could have chosen a dress with accessories to go with the dress at the same time and avoid all this extra work. I went shopping for the accessories I needed then I went to the beauty salon to style my hair.

When I got home to my surprise my niece was there and between the whole crew, including my husband, they got extra busy. My husband was very involved with my oldest son and his family. The young people had a lot to talk about, so I chalked it up to them not having seen each other for some time even though they talked constantly over social media.

It was not until I reflected that I realized they were finalizing and coordinating a surprise for me. I could not tell them about my surprise, not now, it had to wait as everyone was excited to see each other.

Reflections

Why does a God of love allow one to suffer?

_____

_____

_____

How should one react having received a cancer diagnosis?

_____

_____

_____

Who would you consider sharing the diagnosis with?

_____

_____

_____

_____

Chapter 5: The Surprise Party

On February 10th, 2018 was my big dinner outing and everyone was busy getting ready. My husband, George and my son, Malik Anthony left the house early and when they returned George got himself ready. He wore a dark gray Nehru cut suit, white silk shirt and a black bow tie. He then left with my son again said he would return shortly to get me. I got myself together and my daughter and niece insisted on working on my makeup.

We were all ready at about 2:49 pm, just then the phone rang, and it was George letting me know that he was outside waiting for me as our reservation was for 3:00 pm. I mustered up energy to add the finishing touches to my hair and face. The girls also finished up their hair and make-up and we all left the house at 2:55 pm.

I kept asking which restaurant they were taking me to but they would not give me an answer. Shortly after George pulled up to a nondescript building with balloons in the windows and at the main entrance black and gold ribbons and balloons. We all exited the car and walked into the vestibule and then through another door and then I heard everyone shout out SURPRISE !! and when I looked around, I saw family members, longtime friends, my church colleagues, church friends, and cousins whom I had not seen for years. The room was beautifully decorated, and I was left with my mouth opened. I went around to the different tables greeting people and thanking them for this surprise and just enjoying their company. I was incredibly happy to see everyone and most of all I forgot for a moment what I was about to face and in the same breath thanking God for family and friends.

The musician played some good oldies from the 70's and when I finally sat at the Dais table, I was happy and in awe as to how they had pulled this off without me even suspecting anything.

The Deacon prayed over this celebration and blessed the food. We ate, danced, made speeches. I cut my beautiful birthday cake, and everyone was given the opportunity to visit the dessert table to select from the assortment of chocolates and candy they liked including boxed, sliced birthday cake.

At 7 p.m. Everyone departed and my only wish was that the celebration could last longer. Unfortunately, the Banquet Hall had another function scheduled for 8:30 pm. It was an enjoyable evening, and I thanked my family. I knew deep down inside there was another surprise waiting for me and that surprise needed me to be aligned with God so that I could lean on him knowing that he would have my back and his will would prevail one way or the other.

The birthday celebration was over now. I had to prepare myself for my Sunday evening concert. My daughter had purchased tickets for George, herself and I. We were looking forward to enjoying great music and dinner after.

What a way to celebrate my birthday and Valentine's Day. Beautiful music, good company and dining despite what was to come I was truly blessed. Morning mass then followed by the evening outing to Carnegie Hall to see the famous jazz singer, Gregory Porter.

Reflections

Chapter 6: Phase 1 and 2 Action Plans

On February 6, 2018, I had seen my gynecologist. He conducted a physical examination, pap smear, biopsy and the following day a sonogram. My doctor told me then that he suspected cancer but that the results would confirm his suspicion and on February 13, 2018, it was definite that I was facing a battle with Endometrial Cancer.

He immediately referred me to three top Gynecological Oncologist working out of the University hospital in that community. The lead specialist scheduled me for consultation on March 19, 2018, my doctor could then release all medical records that would give the specialist enough time to go over my test results, analyze the data then confirm the stage of cancer and formulate a strategy to attack the cancer to result in a favorable outcome. After consultation a series of examinations were scheduled for my pre-admission tests which would give the surgeon clearance to proceed with a total hysterectomy.

I was told that at my age I did not have to worry about saving my ovaries and that it was best that a total hysterectomy be done.

The date of surgery was set for April 19th, 2018. Following are the tests I had to complete before I could be cleared for surgery:

- March 27, 2018 Cat Scan and chest X-ray
- March 29, 2018 Pre-admission testing
- April 4, 2018 Bilateral Mammogram and Sonogram
- April 6, 2018 Consult with Heart Specialist
- April 10, 2018 Stress Test
- April 11, 2018 Carotid Test
- April 16, 2018 Aorta Test
- Medical clearance sent to Surgeon and Hospital
- April 19, 2018 Admitted for surgery at the University Hospital
- April 26, 2018 Return to doctor's office to check incision and the healing process.
- Rest and nourishment was to continue until May 2, 2018
- Then May 2, 2018 for consult and post-surgery discussion.
- May 18, 2018 Post Operation examination where phase 2 of my treatment was scheduled.

The doctor, of course reiterated the importance of following through with the second phase of treatment. He informed me that he will be prescribing six sessions of Chemotherapy, each session three weeks apart to give my body a chance to rebuild cells and my immune system to recover enough to tolerate safely each session. My start date for Chemotherapy was June 21, 2018, so I had a few weeks to prepare and plan for my care before the first session began.

My husband stayed with me until this consultation and then he returned to secure our summer home. He flew back to New York on May 24, 2018, in time for the oldest granddaughter's graduation from Drexel University and for the start of my chemotherapy.

Reflections

What would you do to move forward with your scheduled plans after receiving life altering news?

_____

_____

_____

_____

How would you have applied Ephesians 6: vs 16-18 to this situation?

_____

_____

_____

_____

What other Bible verses would you lean on for courage?

Lord, the Tiger in My Tank is Cancer

Chapter 7: Obtaining a Support System and Seeking Spiritual Counsel

Knowing that George had to return to Florida as he had been in New York since the beginning of February and now it was the end of April I had to think about a team of family and friends who would be available to support me during each of the chemotherapy sessions whenever George could not be present.

My daughter decided that she would take some time off her busy schedule as long as she had no tour dates. She would fly into New York and accompany me on a few of the chemotherapy sessions.

I still needed others to pick up at least two of the sessions, so I called three of my closet church friends and invited them to lunch. After some discussion we settled on a date and place of their choice which was Red Lobster in Long Island.

It was a drab looking spring day when we met at Red Lobster at about 11:30 am.

We were seated by the host, and we preceded to order our meal. Having completed this, I explained to them why I had summoned them to this emergency lunch meeting. Now Dianne was the Pediatric Nurse, Kamala was the Adolescent behavior therapist and Marlyn was the Home Engineer and volunteer. I was the Sociologist, health educator and Youth guidance counselor to them.

Over the years I had given counsel to the Youths in our Youth Program and to the parents as they navigated their sons high school career and their education path. They could always count on me for guidance and so I knew that I could count on them for at least support throughout this crisis I was facing. I explained to them what I was facing, what my diagnosis was and in what capacity I would need their support. Prayers being one and the other was could I call and count on them to get me to my treatment. That meant take me to the infusion center, stay with me throughout the process and bring me back home.

They all said that I could count on them should the need arise. That load having been lifted off my shoulder we settled in and enjoyed our lunch.

I promised to give them advance notice when the need for their support presented itself, but prayers and encouragement was what I needed most from them.

Having established a support system, I thanked God for placing people in my life that would come to my rescue when it was needed. I now had to prepare myself spiritually to start the battle ahead of me that battle would begin on June 21, 2018.

I sought out my Pastor for spiritual counsel and I explained to him what I was about to face. He prayed with me, anointed me, prayed with me again, gave me his blessings and reassured me that all was well and that I should continue to trust in God and on his promise to deliver me and in his time, all would be done according to his word. All I had to do was ask for his deliverance trust and believe.

Reflections

How would you, the reader, encourage the author to seek support during this precarious period of her life?

_____

_____

_____

_____

What do you think accounted for the author's strength in going through the chemo-therapy process?

_____

_____

_____

_____

Chapter 8 - The First Visit To The Infusion Center

George accompanied me on my first visit to the Infusion center. I had to be there for 8:00 am on the morning of June 21, 2018. When I arrived, I had to check in at the reception intake desk. I then sat in the waiting area and in about ten minutes a nurse came and escorted my husband and I to the area where the chemo would be administered. A technician took my blood and rushed it to their lab. Even though they had taken blood 5 days prior to the first treatment the nurse explained that each time I reported for treatment they will be taking blood to make sure that my platelets did not fall to where it would be detrimental to me for them to proceed with treatment.

After about fifteen minutes the technician came back with the report. The nurse proceeded to set up the intravenous equipment in my arm and added the first medication. The nurse then brought a warm blanket and covered me. The first medication would run for one hour. My husband was given a chair and he was directed to the kitchen area where he could get tea or coffee while he waited with me. He was also encouraged to bring me tea as that would also help to keep me warm.

The nurse checked on me periodically and when the timer went off after an hour, she came over to me and added the second medicine and that too would run for another hour and ten minutes and again the timer was set. The nurse then gave me a menu where I could select lunch for my husband and I as long as the meal fell into a set price range. If it went over the set price I would be responsible for the difference.

I ordered a tuna salad sandwich and George ordered a bowl of their hearty soup and at noon the order was delivered to us. Surprisingly I ate but during my eating the nurse had to add another medication and she warned me that I would feel sleepy, and do you know before I could finish my delicious sandwich, I fell asleep. The nurse wanted me to eat a meal while I was there, I guess to make sure I did eat a meal before I went home.

I must have slept for a little over an hour for when I opened my eyes, I had to go to the bathroom. The nurse unplugged the IV pole so that I could wheel it to the bathroom and when I returned, she helped me back into my chair and she gave me a fresh warm blanket.

Shortly after this she added another medication and told me that I was coming to the end of my treatment for today and that I only had another 40 minutes left in my treatment.

I finished my sandwich along with a cup of tea. I remained in the chair until the nurse came over and removed the IV from my arm. I rested for a few minutes until I felt that I was able to get up and walk on my own without feeling lightheaded.

I was then discharged home and instructed to drink a lot of water or clear liquid and to rest whenever I felt tired. I was also told to add additional salt and spices to my meals as I would not have any taste in my mouth. It was important that I eat a well-balanced meal each day. I was also advised to continue my vitamin regime.

I received therapy for the duration of eighteen weeks comprising of 6 sessions, each session three-weeks apart and it ended on September 7, 2018. Each time I went for chemotherapy I had to go through the same routine and each time it got more difficult for them to draw blood. The doctor encouraged me to have a port installed on my upper chest, but I did not want to go through that procedure, after all I had had major surgery, I did not want to expose myself to any infection and I did not think I could tolerate walking around with a tube implanted in my chest.

I persevered and between my family and friends I completed the chemo treatment, and they sure did not let me sit around and feel sorry for myself. They encouraged me to take short walks, to dress up and go to church, go to the supermarket to get needed fruit and vegetables and lots of alkaline water. I set up a routine of prayers for every morning and evening.

My son made himself available to take me to the additional appointments including the taking of blood one week prior to each chemotherapy treatment. It is important to note that the infusion center that administered the treatment gave me a printout of my blood work so that I could monitor how my blood and immune system reacted to the therapy. It was a gauge to see if I was at risk for hospitalization and whether my blood platelets were recovering in the three weeks span in between each treatment.

It lasted eighteen weeks. The only traumatic experience I faced was the total loss of my hair after the first treatment. Yes! I went bald.

I had my daughter cut the hanging matted hair off and my husband shaved my head. I was devastated I loved my soft curly hair, and I am not ashamed to say I cried for days.

I owe my tolerance, attitude, fortitude, faith and strength all to God Almighty because he was with me before each treatment and after each treatment along with the wrapping of myself in the 23rd Psalm, reading GOD'S Medicine, I was lifted out of the fire and came through this phase triumphantly. All Glory, honor and praise be to God Almighty.

Reflections

Chapter 9 - Phase 3 and Final Stage of Treatment

That was not the end on September 19, 2018 I was scheduled for a CT scan of the abdomen and pelvic area, I was worried because I did not know which way the result of the test would go. I waited and prayed for a good outcome. When the results came back, I was happy. There was some scar tissue but with time that would disappear. Now I could prepare myself for the final stage of treatment. I had to visit the doctor to be examined and to go over all that I had gone through to date.

I was hoping that with the CT scan result and blood work my doctor would say that I did not have to take the radiation. Well, I was disappointed because guess what? I had to go through the radiation phase.

My doctor explained to me that the goal was to give me everything necessary to not have the cancer return and that was the best way he knew how to have a good outcome for me. As disappointed as I was; I told him to go ahead and set up treatment. He referred me to one of his colleagues who was the best in radiation therapy treatment and the treatment center was located in the same hospital that performed my hysterectomy it was a place that I felt safe in so, I reviewed the schedule set up for me.

So now another hurdle to surmount, that of radiation. The radiation treatment would be dispensed in two phases for a total of 25 treatments over a period of five weeks. This meant that I had to report to the hospital's radiation department every day from Monday to Friday at 8:00 am each morning.

I would then be placed in a machine for 15 to 20 minutes each day. I experienced side effects for the first three weeks. I was tired, constipated, suffered bladder irritation and some anal irritation. For the irritation I was prescribed Aquaphor cream and a mild laxative for the constipation.

After the five weeks of treatment was over, I entered phase two of the radiation that comprised of a short break of one week followed by the cylinder treatment.

This treatment was three visits, once weekly for eight to twelve minutes of the radioactive seed insert.

Having completed those visits, I was fitted for a Vaginal dilator. Two weeks later I returned to the radiation center for an examination where I was shown how to use the dilator. I was to perform this therapy three times weekly and each treatment was to last ten minutes for the duration of one year. I was to make follow up visits to the radiation doctor once every three months following seeing the Gynecological Oncologist.

Overall, I was to be followed by these two doctors for the next three years during which time the therapy would decrease each following year to twice per week and in the final year once per week. My visits to the Gynecological Oncologist would be once every three months in the first year then once every four months, then once every six months and lastly to conclude once per year in the last year.

At that point I could say that I have successfully completed the treatments and that I am now cancer free.

I am at the point now where my therapy is once per week, but I am hoping that when I see the doctor again, he will say that I can now see him once every six months for the rest of this year trusting that at the end of the year I can go back to a regular once per year doctor's office visit. To date I feel good, but one never knows what is happening with what one cannot see. I leave that up to God and the doctors in whose care he placed me in. I must add that during this ordeal I lost my primary care physician to retirement.

I am sad because I needed her to guide me to the end of this journey. She had guided me through twenty- eight years of keeping me on track with my medical needs and I do not know where to start trying to find a new doctor. They sure do not make those kinds of doctors anymore. I am most grateful for her care and guidance through the most crucial period of my life, and I pray that God will guide me to find a Primary care doctor to fill her shoe.

Reflections

What lessons can we learn from the woman with the issue of blood in the bible.?

_____

_____

_____

_____

_____

Do you think that the author's faith brought her through? Explain.

_____

_____

_____

_____

_____

_____

Did the author consider herself an outcast and allowed it to dictate the outcome of her future blessings?

_____

_____

_____

_____

_____

_____

_____

_____

_____

_____

_____

_____

Chapter 10 - Medications and Other Aids

Rejoice Always. Pray without ceasing. In all circumstances give thanks, for this is the will of God for you in Christ Jesus.
Thessalonians 5:16-18

Following find a list of some of the medications that I was given intravenously and I will list some of their effects on my body.

The first medication I received was Taxol. Its generic name is Paclitaxel, it is an anti-cancer chemotherapy drug classified as a "plant alkaloid". It is an irritant which causes inflammation of the vein so the nurse or doctor who administers it must be carefully trained because if this medication escapes from the vein it can cause tissue damage. It does not come in a pill form.

Some of the side effects are low blood counts, risk for infection, anemia and/or bleeding, hair loss, pain in the joints and muscles, peripheral neuropathy, nausea and vomiting, diarrhea, swelling of feet or ankles, low blood pressure, nail changes, etc. Note these side effects return to normal once treatment is over.

The other major medication given was Carboplatin. Carboplatin is an anticancer drug ("antineoplastic" or "cytotoxic") it is classified as an alkylating agent. It is used to treat other types of cancer as a preparation for stem cell or bone marrow transplant. This is also given by infusion into a vein or directly into the peritoneal cavity in the abdomen. The amount given depends on height, weight and your general health.

Some of the side effects are low blood count, Nausea and vomiting, taste change, hair loss, weakness, abnormal magnesium level, abdominal pain, diarrhea, constipation, decreased sensation numbness and tingling of the extremities, sensory loss and difficulty walking, fever of 100.4F, chest pain and difficulty breathing require that you contact the doctor immediately. These symptoms become progressively more severe, with continued treatment.

To help to alleviate some of these symptoms it is suggested that you drink a lot of water up to three quarts within every 24 hours, use of a soft toothbrush and rinse your mouth at least three times a day with baking soda, salt and water mixture and of course avoid sun exposure and wear at least SPF 15 or higher sunblock and also get plenty of rest.

I was blessed in that I did not experience most of the symptoms I was told to watch out for, and I think that it was because I followed my doctor's advice to the letter.

This information is just a tip of the iceberg you will have to read the scientific journal on cancer to see how the chemotherapy kills cells and halt cell division and at the same time damage the RNA or DNA that tells the cell how to copy itself.

It is imperative that we as women pay attention to the cues our body gives us and report this to the doctors this way, they can refer you to a specialists who can best investigate and consult with your primary care doctor so that a viable plan of care that would give you the best chance to survive and live with cancer.

Taking care of our bodies with the right nutrients can also give you the edge in surviving cancer. My whole diet changed, and I am currently on an adventure trying what foods work to keep body with a strong immune system because that will make the difference in surviving the battle.

It is my hope that this book serves as a guidance for all who walked with me on this journey that is not quite yet over, but I trust that God has a plan for me that is why he has brought me thus far.

Ways To Learn More

National Oral Health Information Clearinghouse
Call 1-866-232-4528
Visit http://www.nidcr.nih.gov

National Cancer Institute
http://www.smokefree.gov
Call 1-800-4-CANCER 1-800-422-6237

American Cancer Society
1-800-ACS-2345 or 1-800-227-2345

Cancer Support Community
Dedicated to providing support, education and hope to people affected by cancer.
Call 1-888-793-9355 or 202-659-9709

Cancer Care. Inc.
Offers free support, information, financial assistance, and practical help to people with Cancer and their loved ones.
Call 1-800-813-HOPE (1-800-813-4673)
E-mail: info@CancerCare.org

Food Suggestions

Some food suggested to eat during the chemotherapy and radiation if you did not feel like eating were as follows:

Liquid Foods
Soups
Bouillon
Broth
Strained soup
Tomato Soup
Soup with pureed potatoes

Drinks
Carbonated beverages
Coffee
Eggnog (pasteurized and Alcohol free)
Fruit drinks, juices, Fruit punch
Milk, Milkshakes, Smoothies
Sports drink, Tea
Tomato juice, vegetable juice
Water

Fats
Butter
Cream
Margarine
Oil
Sour Cream

Sweets
Custard (soft or baked)
Frozen Yogurt (plain or vanilla)
Fruit purees that are watered down
Gelatin
Honey
Plain ice cream
Ice milk
Jelly
Pudding
Syrup

Replacements
Instant breakfast drinks
Supplements
Liquid meal replacements

High Fiber Foods
Foods that may help if you have constipation.
Bran muffins
Bran or whole-grain cereals
Brown or wild rice
Cooked dry peas and beans
Whole-wheat bread
Whole-wheat pastas
Fresh fruit
Dried fruit, such as apricots, dates, prunes
Vegetables
Fresh fruit
Raw or cooked vegetables, such as broccoli corn, green beans, karela, spinach

Snacks
Granola
Nuts
Popcorn
Sunflower seeds
Trail mix

Low-Fiber Foods

This list may help if you have diarrhea.

Chicken or turkey (skinless)
Cooked refined cereals
Cottage cheese, eggs, fish
Noodles, potatoes (baked or mashed)
White bread, white rice
Asparagus
Bananas
Canned fruit
Peaches
Pears
Applesauce
Clear fruit juice
Vegetable juice

Snacks

Angel food cake
Gelatin, Sherbet or sorbet
Saltine crackers
Yogurt (plain or vanilla)

In addition, I personally used wheat grass in my shakes and Ribena in my alkaline water and glucose as a sweetener instead of sugar.

References That Helped Me on This Journey

God's Medicine by Kenneth E. Hagin

Thought Conditioners by Norman Vincent Peale

My Saint Pio Prayer Book (A Treasury of Prayers from (Padre Pio Foundation of America)

Faith in the Valley by Iyanla Vanzant

A Call to Joy by Matthew Kelly

The Holy Bible (The New American Version)

Finding New Life in the Spirit by Lawrence A Gollner, Leo A Pursley, D.D.

The Truth about Cancer by Ty M. Bollenger, Hay house, Inc. Printed USA, 1st Edition, October 2016

The Cancer Survivor's Guide: Foods That Help You Fight Back by Neal D Barnard, MD, Jennifer K Reilly, RD (Healthy Living Publications)

Summer Town, TN 38483, Printed in Canada 2008

www.ingramcontent.com/pod-product-compliance
Lightning Source LLC
Chambersburg PA
CBHW070817220526
45466CB00002B/697